PROVEN WAYS TO TREAT UTI

Understanding the causes, symptoms, effects and treatment of UTI

By

Dr DOUGLAS JASON

Copyright © (DR DOUGLAS JASON) 2023. All rights reserved

Before this document is duplicated or reproduced in any manner, the publisher's consent must be gained.

Therefore, the contents within can neither be stored electronically, transferred, nor kept in a database. Neither in part nor in full can the document be copied, scanned, faxed, or retained without approval from the publisher or creator.

TABLE OF CONTENT

ABOUT THE AUTHOR

INTRODUCTION

TABLE OF CONTENTS

PROVEN WAYS TO TREAT UTI

Understanding the causes, symptoms, effects and treatment of UTI

INTRODUCTION

CHAPTER 1
What Are the Symptoms of a UTI?

CHAPTER 2
Who Is at Risk of UTI Complications?

CHAPTER 3
UTI vs. STD

CHAPTER 4

Honeymoon Cystitis

CHAPTER 5
Stealth UTI

CHAPTER 6
Possible UTI Complications

CHAPTER 7
Causes of Urinary Tract Infection

CHAPTER 8
Symptoms of Urinary Tract Infection in Men.

CHAPTER 9
How to Treat a Urinary Tract Infection(UTIs)

CHAPTER 10

How to Prevent and Treat Recurrent UTIs

CHAPTER 11
Nursing Homes and Hospitals' UTI Risk.

CHAPTER 12
How Does Urinary Tract Infection Affect the Elderly?

CHAPTER 13
How Does Infant Urinary Tract Infection Affect Them?

CHAPTER 14
Toddler UTI or Accident During Potty Training?

CHAPTER 15

How to Prevent Urinary Tract Infections

ABOUT THE AUTHOR

Dr. Douglas Jason is a certified dietician who has a strong passion for wellness and a big eagerness to help people all over the world. He uses healthy food, herbs, spices, and other useful tools to help mankind realize its overall goal of optimum health.

INTRODUCTION

WHAT IS A URINARY TRACT INFECTION.
When a pathogen infects one or more urinary system organs (kidneys, ureters, bladder, or urethra), it results in a urinary tract infection (UTI) (most frequently, bacteria). About 50% of all females will experience a UTI at some point in their lifetime. Many UTIs are not dangerous, but if the infection spreads to the kidneys, it can cause significant sickness and even death.

CHAPTER 1

What Are the Symptoms of a UTI?

infected bladder.

Most UTIs are relatively common bladder infections. Although some people may experience little or no symptoms, the typical bladder infection symptoms include dysuria (pain or burning during urinating), low abdomen pain, and/or murky, unpleasant-smelling, or unusual-smelling urine.

kidney infection

Some bladder infections worsen when the bacteria advance (retrograde) the ureters to the kidneys, failing to resolve. In addition to the symptoms listed for bladder infections on the preceding slide, other symptoms include lower back discomfort (flank pain on one or both sides), fever, chills, and nausea and/or vomiting are frequently present.

CHAPTER 2

Who Is at Risk of UTI Complications?

The following people are at a higher risk for UTI consequences, such as infection spread to the kidneys or elsewhere in the body, even though a bladder infection is not a medical emergency:

expecting mothers
individuals with diabetes
those who suffer from renal issues like kidney stones or obstructions
people in their 80s
Immune-deficient individuals
enlarged prostates in males
those who have indwelling catheters or urinary retention

CHAPTER 3

UTI vs. STD

The symptoms of other very frequent forms of infections, such as sexually transmitted diseases, may resemble those of UTIs as detailed in the preceding slides (STDs).

These illnesses include trichomoniasis, chlamydia, and gonorrhea (and occasionally syphilis as well). To identify and distinguish between an STD and a UTI, lab testing is easily accessible. Although it is not typically present in UTIs, the discharge of pus or fluid from the penis or vagina is a sign frequently found in STDs.

CHAPTER 4

Honeymoon Cystitis

The phrase for a UTI that frequently happens after sexual activity is "honeymoon cystitis." After sexual activity, some women regularly develop UTIs (honeymoon or not). The urethra can become infected as a result of sexual activity pushing harmful bacteria into the area. UTIs are more common in women who have had a diaphragm implanted for birth control. For the treatment of honeymoon cystitis, antibiotics are employed.

CHAPTER 5

Stealth UTI

UTIs without symptoms are common; the condition is known as asymptomatic bacteriuria and urine testing can reveal the presence of bacteria in the urine. Typically, this illness is not treated, however in some patients, antibiotics are preferable (for example, pregnant women, some children, and kidney transplant patients).

CHAPTER 6

Possible UTI Complications

UTIs can lead to two main problems. The first is an infection that has progressed to either one kidney or both. Renal function may be harmed if the infection persists, which might lead to kidney failure or total loss of kidney function.

The second issue is that the infectious agents might sporadically reach the bloodstream, where they may spread to other organs or, extremely infrequently, resulting in sepsis and death.

CHAPTER 7

Causes of Urinary Tract Infection

Most UTIs begin when pathogens, typically bacteria like E. coli, enter the urethra and proceed retrogradely (upward) to the bladder. Up until the distal urethra, urine is often sterile.

Women have shorter urethras than men, and most doctors believe that this is a major factor in why women experience more UTIs than men.

Who Has the Highest Urinary Tract Infection (UTI) Risk?

The following additional risk factors exist in addition to those already mentioned, such as being an older or immunocompromised person or a woman who engages in sexual activity:

not enough liquids consumed (slows the wash of pathogens out of the body)

Frequently bathing (soaking in a fluid that may promote retrograde infections)
awaiting urination (promotes retrograde bacterial movement)
renal stones (causes slowing or partial blockage of urine flow)
Solutions For Health From Our Sponsors

CHAPTER 8

Symptoms of Urinary Tract Infection in Men.

Adult males rarely have UTIs; when they do, there is typically an underlying cause (for example, having an enlarged prostate or kidney stone or being an elderly person with a catheter).

Methods for Urinary Tract Infection Testing (UTIs)

After a patient provides their medical history and undergoes a physical examination, a urinalysis is typically the next diagnostic procedure performed. The test reveals whether germs, white and red blood cells and chemical abnormalities are present. It can suggest that additional investigations, such as urine cultures and tests for bacterial medication susceptibility, are necessary. Even though it is possible to do easy tests at home, such as the pee dipstick test, they are not entirely reliable. It is essential to have your doctor assess your symptoms and the findings of your urine test.

CHAPTER 9

How to Treat a Urinary Tract Infection(UTIs)

Most UTIs (and many mild-to-moderate kidney infections) are treated with oral antibiotics, although severe kidney infections are frequently treated in hospitals with IV antibiotics.

To identify the pathogens and assess their antibiotic resistance, several doctors are providing urine samples. Due to antibiotic resistance, it is common for a doctor to call a patient and switch antibiotics. To flush bacteria out of the urinary tract, the doctor would typically advise the patient to drink enough fluids (water) and to urinate frequently.

CHAPTER 10

How to Prevent and Treat Recurrent UTIs

Recurrent UTIs are not unusual, but if you experience three or more UTIs annually, you should ask your primary care physician (PCP) for a referral to a urologist to rule out any underlying urinary tract issues that might be the reason. Additionally, your PCP could advise taking an oral antibiotic after having sex or taking an oral antibiotic as needed if you get UTI symptoms.

Diabetes vs. UTI

Diabetes increases the risk of urinary tract infections (UTIs) because diabetes can induce high urine sugar levels, which provide a favorable environment for bacterial development. Diabetes patients frequently have immune systems that are less effective at fighting infections. Diabetes damage to the nerves can lead to insufficient emptying of the bladder, which promotes bacterial survival and retrograde infections.

Pregnancy vs. UTI

Due to hormonal changes that may affect regular urinary tract function and the enlarging uterus' potential to put pressure on the bladder and ureters, pregnancy raises the risk of UTIs. The result is a slowing of urine production and a holding or delaying of urination in pregnant women. As a result, germs can thrive well in these settings. If you suspect you have a UTI while pregnant, you should let your doctor (or doctors) know because UTIs may contribute to preterm labor.

Menopause and UTIs
Elevated estrogen levels after menopause. Because estrogen offers some degree of protection against UTIs, some women may become more vulnerable to UTIs as a result of its decline following menopause.

CHAPTER 11

Nursing Homes and Hospitals' UTI Risk.

Many people need catheters because they can't get up to use the restroom while they're in the hospital (a tube put through the urethra into the bladder to allow urine to flow). In certain people, the catheter and the area around it are entry points for bacteria into the bladder. People who have lengthy hospital stays or who are in long-term care facilities like nursing homes are more likely to experience this issue. Elderly UTIs pose a major issue.

30

CHAPTER 12

How Does Urinary Tract Infection Affect the Elderly?

Both men and women develop UTIs in the elderly. Even though they may experience typical UTI symptoms, elderly people frequently experience other UTI symptoms. Only agitation, delirium, confusion, and/or behavioral problems may be all that they display. Elderly people are more likely to get complications like kidney infections or sepsis from UTIs.

CHAPTER 13

How Does Infant Urinary Tract Infection Affect Them?

It's a good idea to change a child's wet or dirty diaper to help avoid UTIs. Additionally, wiping from front to back lowers the risk of having UTIs in both males and females. Infants and young children can experience the same classic UTI symptoms as the elderly, but they are unable to tell anyone they are experiencing them. Fever, strange-smelling urine, decreased appetite, vomiting, abdominal discomfort, and fussy behavior are all indications of a UTI in children. Kidney damage can be avoided in children by treating UTIs quickly.

How Does Children's Urinary Tract Infection Affect Them?

Before puberty, UTIs affect 3% of girls and 1% of boys. Some of these kids have anatomical issues with their urinary systems, which make retrograde flow possible and provide bacteria with an easy pathway to the kidneys. For diagnosis and therapy, it is typical to consult a pediatric urologist. Other kids might put off going potty, and some might not be able to fully unwind their muscles to empty their bladders. Increased fluid intake and promoting more potty visits may be beneficial for these kids.

CHAPTER 14

Toddler UTI or Accident During Potty Training?

Potty training a child can be challenging (and the adults). Accidents, however, are a necessary part of this training, so adults should be prepared for them, and kids should learn that they can happen and not to be upset if they do. Some kids resist potty training by yelling and sobbing. While reassurance is helpful, not all kids can be trained to use the toilet by a certain age. It's possible that some kids aren't quite ready for training when other kids are. Children frequently mimic the actions of other kids. For many kids, watching a sibling their age or a daycare friend successfully use the restroom has been helpful. The refusal of a youngster to participate in potty training is not typically interpreted as a UTI indication.

CHAPTER 15

How to Prevent Urinary Tract Infections

The prevention of UTIs has been discussed in the slides that came before; the following is a brief list of typical and simple techniques to do so:

daily large amounts of water
Don't "delay" urinating by postponing using the restroom.
From front to back, wipe
Avoid using feminine care sprays.
Showers are preferable to baths.

Cranberry juice for infections of the urinary tract Cranberry juice may help prevent UTIs, according to several studies because there is some evidence that it prevents E. coli from adhering to the bladder wall. Tablets or pills made with cranberries could potentially achieve this. But there isn't any solid proof that cranberries, in any form, help treat a UTI. Before using cranberry products to prevent UTIs, those with a history of kidney stones should consult their doctor(s).

www.ingramcontent.com/pod-product-compliance
Lightning Source LLC
Chambersburg PA
CBHW050323220526
45465CB00005B/2105